Thank you for choosing The Fat-Burning Ultimate Workout System for People Over 40

Consult your physician before starting this program.

By voluntarily following my program you acknowledge, and agreed to a liability waiver and release Paolo Nana for any responsibility.

The Benefits of This Program

Body Fat Reduction.

Lean Mass Gain (muscles).

Obesity Prevention.

Reduce Hunger.

Reduce Insulin Resistance.

Prevent /Reverse Type 2 Diabetes.

Blood Sugar Will Improve.

Blood Pressure Will Improve.

Cholesterol Quality Will Improve.

Reduce Inflammation in the body.

May safeguard brain function.

May Reduce Risk of Cancer.

And many more benefits.

CONTENT

1. Nutrition.

2. Daily Weight Management Log

3. Muscles target.

4. Training technique.

5. Workout Log.

6. Progress Report.

<u>WHO</u> should start this program? Individuals that are already familiar with weight training and wish to improve their physical shape and overall health.

<u>FREQUENCY</u> 3/4/5/6 sessions per week. Choose the one that fits you beast.

<u>MUSCLES TARGETED</u>: Back, Chest, Shoulder, Biceps, Triceps, Abdominals, Quads, Hamstrings, and Calves.

Aerobic Exercise Option.

Remember, to fully benefit from my system you must follow both, the TRAINING and NUTRITION aspect of the program. Neglecting either one would prevent you to achieve your goal.

CHOSING THE RIGHT FOOD

My intent is to be able you to maintain an eating program that is compatible with your palate. If you don't like the food that you consume, obviously, the diet would be soon abandoned thus you will be again on square one like most people that start a new diet each month.

You need to educate yourself about healthy food. It doesn't mean that you have to have a degree in nutrition, but a general idea regarding the 3 macronutrients (Fat, Protein, and Carbohydrate).

FAT

Fat is the nutrient that we all love, it gives that rich taste to the food, but it comes with a high price; one gram of fat has (9 grams of calories) more than double the number of calories found in protein and carbohydrates (4 gr.).

Stay away from trans-fats; they bring trouble to your health. Recent studies have revealed that *Trans - fats* are harmful because the oil is subjected to a process known as HYDROGENATION that acts as cement in the human heart vascular system.

Consume instead lard, butter, tallow, eggs, olive oil, coconut oil, avocado, olives, ghee, palm oil, avocado oil, fish oil. Nuts and seeds in moderation.

PROTEIN

 I won't put you to sleep with details about protein function in the body. What is important, instead, is to understand the impact that protein has when we exercise. A single muscle fiber consists of amino acids which are the building blocks of muscle protein.

You need to consume the right amount of protein in order to recover from the damage of elastic tissue (protein) that occurs during training. Choose good quality of protein like fish, see-food, meat, eggs, and poultry.

CARBOHYADRATE

Grains (bread, pasta, and rice), sweets, vegetables, and fruits.

You need to know that not all carbohydrates are metabolized at the same rate. Food that has a fast rate of absorption (high glycemic index) will trigger a spike of insulin into the bloodstream causing a vicious sugar craving cycle, and serious health consequences. Gravitate towards carbohydrates that have the lowest glycemic index and rich in fibers, like vegetables.

APPENDIX

As we get older, we do not need to eat too many carbohydrates. By eating fewer carbs and more fat the body uses lipids for energy, which is a healthier source of fuel for our organism. So consider this part of the program more as a lifestyle than a fast fix.

By eating a low carbohydrate diet, the body tends to flash out electrolyze from the body, especially sodium. So, make sure you taking enough sodium to prevent muscle cramps.

SUPPLEMENTS

Real food is always the best, yet supplements may be more convenient when we are on the run. You should look for an established company when buy supplements.

Whey and egg-albumin-protein deliver high quality of essential amino acid for the repair and growth of the muscle tissue.

Multivitamins and minerals should be taken daily. They fight the free radicals (oxidants, the enemy of our health) by delivering antioxidants to the cell.

Creatine is widely used among gym-goers. It improves physical perform by providing energy, muscle contraction, and faster recuperating period.

If you would like to try this supplement, you should avoid the more is the better mentality.

Sometimes, companies sell the product encouraging you to take mega-dose of creatine for the first five days, this high amount of creatine do not translate into higher creatine levels in your muscle. Instead, they may be the very cause of the side effects, including intestinal cramping, diarrhea, increased urination, and dehydration.

To avoid this problem you can try chewable creatine table or the chewing creatine gum. Both give an exact dose of creatine and you don't have to worry about overdosing.

NUTRITION

<u>This part of the program must be followed 100%.</u>

The first step is to establish, <u>proximally</u>, the number of calories you need to consume to reach your goal.

For example, let's say you weigh 200 pounds and want to lose 15 lbs. So your ideal weight would be 185 lbs. Now, you want to know the daily amount of food you need to consume in order to lose those extra pounds. To do so, you have to find out your Basal Metabolism (BM) which is the number of calories your body requires at rest within a period of 24 hours. But to be able to estimate exactly the BM, you have to spend half day in a lab and pay lots money. Instead, you can <u>GENERALLY</u> calculate your BM in others ways; one of these is done by multiplying your <u>TARGETED</u> body-weight by 10.

Example: Targeted weight 185 lbs.

185 by 10 = 1850

1850 is the number of daily calories that you need to consume daily.

Now that you know your calories goal, you have to divide it into macronutrients (carb 1 gram = 4 kcal.) (protein 1gr. = 4 kcal.) (fat 1gr. = 9kcal.).

Because this program is based on LOW CARBS diet, you need to adapt to it gradually.

Here below are 3 tiers.

Tier #1 Low Carbs. (11% of carbs from total calories, 26% Protein, and 63% Fat)
Tier #2 Medium Carbs (16% of carbs from total calories, 26% Protein, 58% Fat)
Tier #3 High Carbs. (22% of carbs from total calories, 26% Protein, 52% Fat)

From the percentage of the calories, now you can figure out the amount of gram you need from macronutrients.

Example: Tier #3 (high carbs)
Daily calories 1850
22% of 1850 = 407 kcal. Divided by 4kcal = 100gr. of carbs.
26% of 1850 = 481kcal. Divided by 4 = 120gr. of protein.
52% of 1850 = 962kcal. Divided by 9 = 107gr. of fat.

I recommend to start with tier #3 and let your body adapt for about three weeks. Then move to tier #2 stay for three weeks, and finally tier #1.

DAILY FOOD LOG

Once you have established your tier, find out the micronutrients and fill the blanks below.

Daily caloric intake: _______

Fat Grams ______

Prot. Grams______

Carbs Grams______

Meals	Fat	Protein	Carbs	Calories
1				
2				
3				
4				

At the end of the day fill the blanks below. The numbers should match the above values.

Total fat___gr.   **Total prot___gr.**   **Total carbs__gr**   **Total Kcal.=**

<u>Make copies</u>

TRAINING

Monday: Chest, Part of the Shoulders, Abs.

Tuesday: Back, Part of the Shoulder, Abs.

Wednesday: Triceps, Biceps, Abs.

Thursday: Legs

Option Friday (Repeat Monday Workout)

Option Saturday (Repeat Tuesday Workout)

<u>Cardio Option</u>: use any cardio pieces of equipments (Treadmills, Bikes, Elliptical, Skiers, etc.). Make sure your heart beats at circa **70% of your VO 2max.**

To <u>approximately</u> estimate your target heart rate subtracts the number of your age from 220 then find the **70%** of the resulted number to establish your anaerobic threshold.

Example:

    You are 40 years old

    220-40= 180

    70% of 180= 126

So, your heart rate should be around 126 beats per minute. Keeping the heart rate too low won't bring any benefit to the cardiovascular workout.

Cardio, 30/45 minutes.

PROGRESS REPORT

Record your progress periodically

Date	Weight	Chest	Waist	Bicep	Thigh

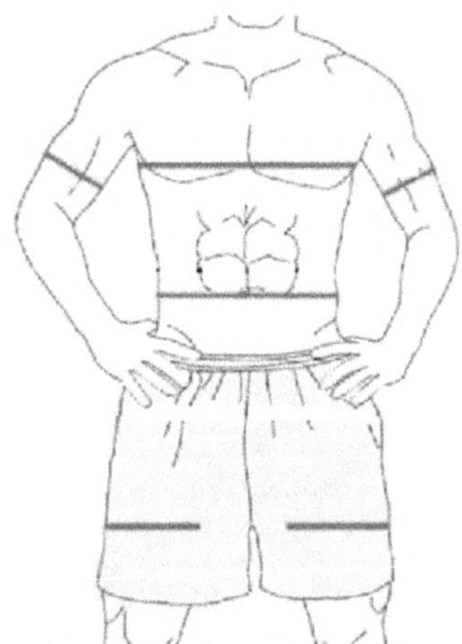

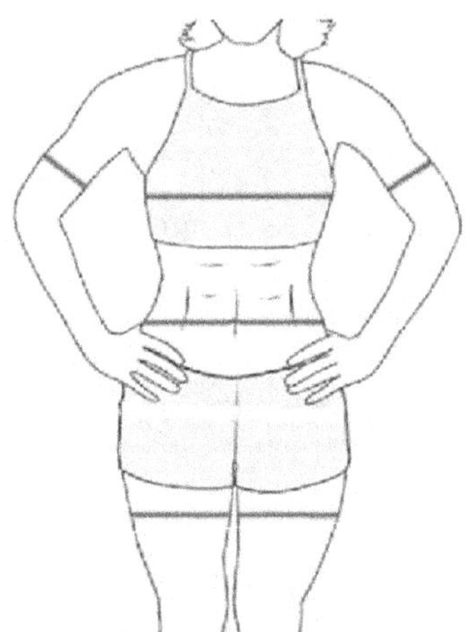

WORKOUT SESSION 1 CHEST & SHOULDERS

CHEST: 4 Exercises / 4 sets / 8 - 10 Reps to Failure.

45/60 Seconds of Rest between Sets

Exercise # 1

Bench or Machine Press

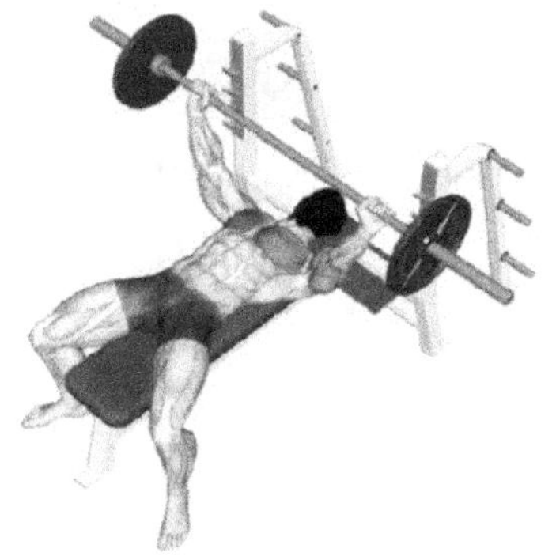

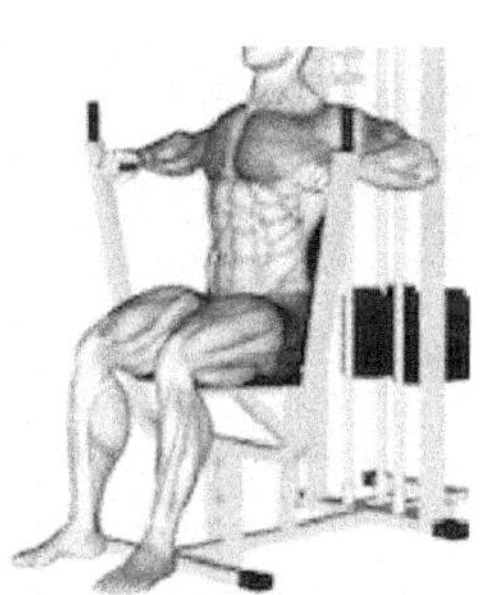

Exercise # 2

Decline Bench, Machine or Low Angle Cable

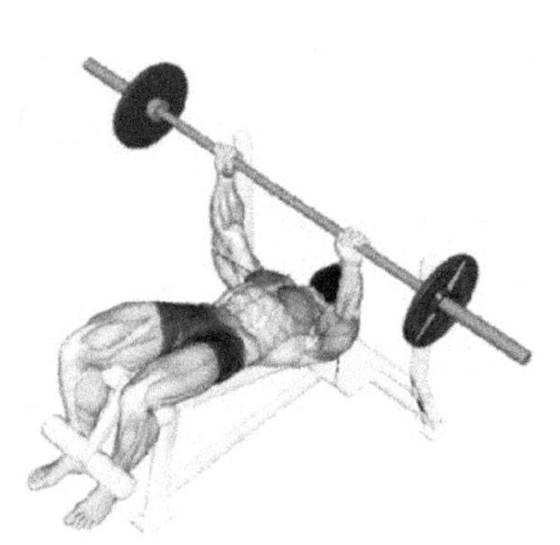

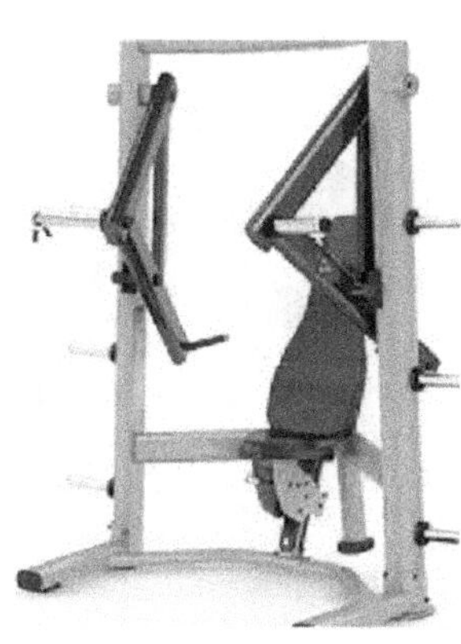

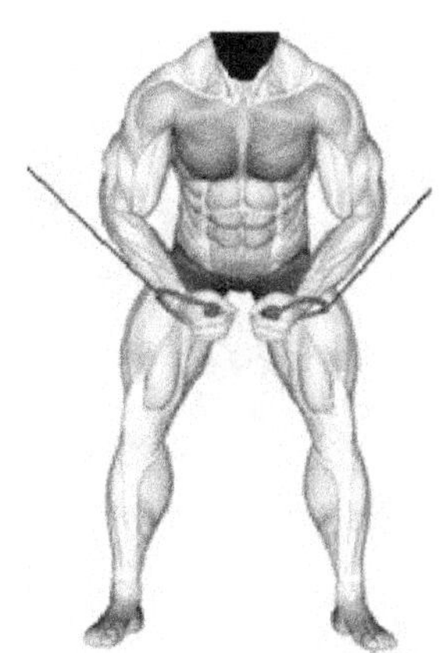

Exercise # 3

Multiple Choices Fly Chest Exercise

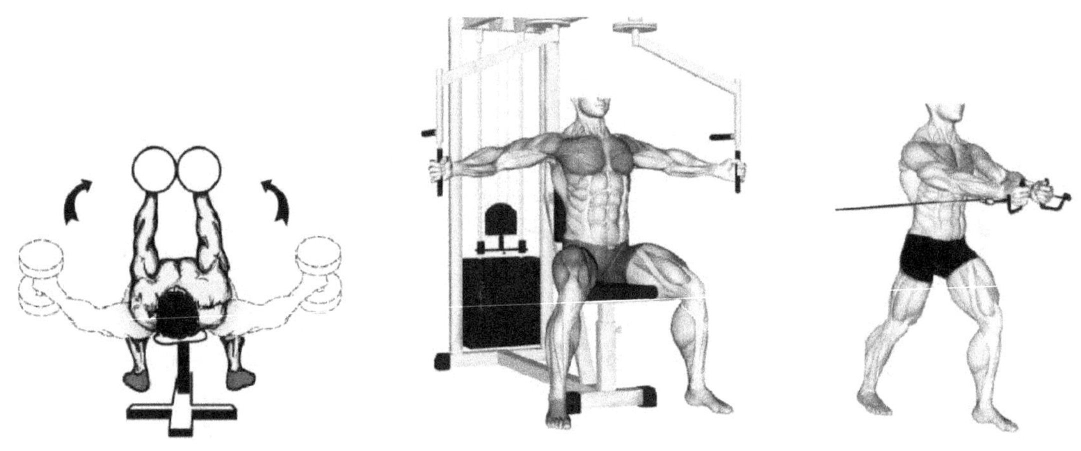

Exercise # 4

Multiple Choices High Chest Exercise

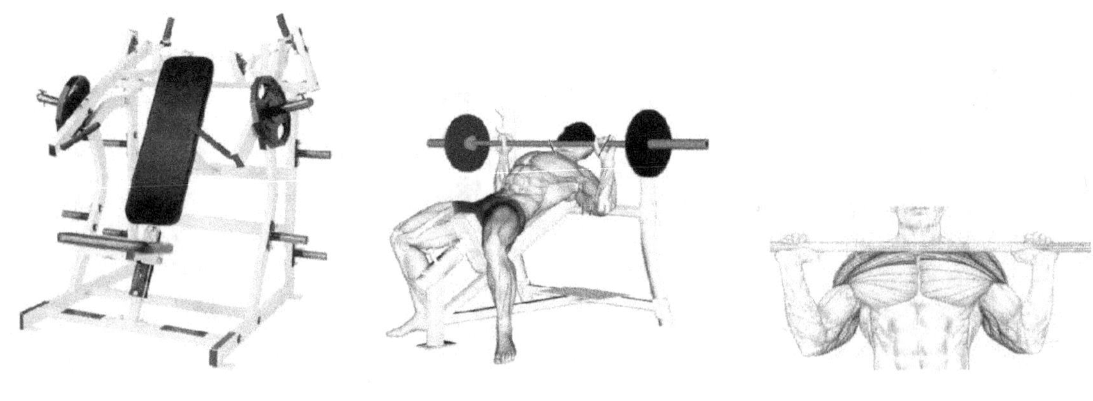

Smith Machine

Exercise # 5

Elbows Squeeze Shoulder Exercise Sequence

1 Exercise, 5 Sets of 10 -12 to Failure

45/60 Seconds of Rest between Sets

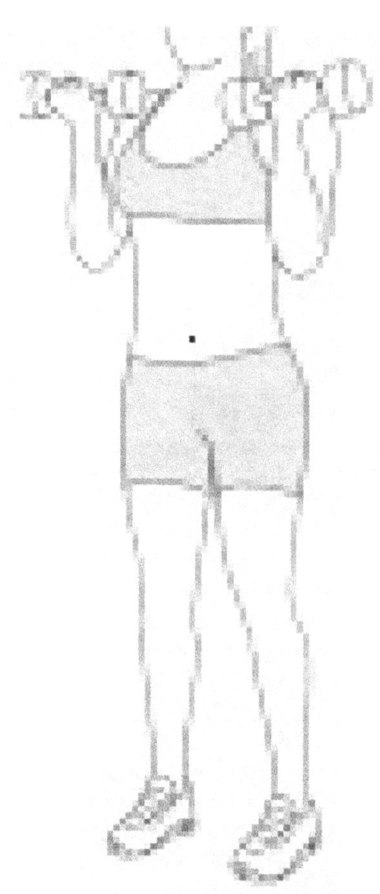
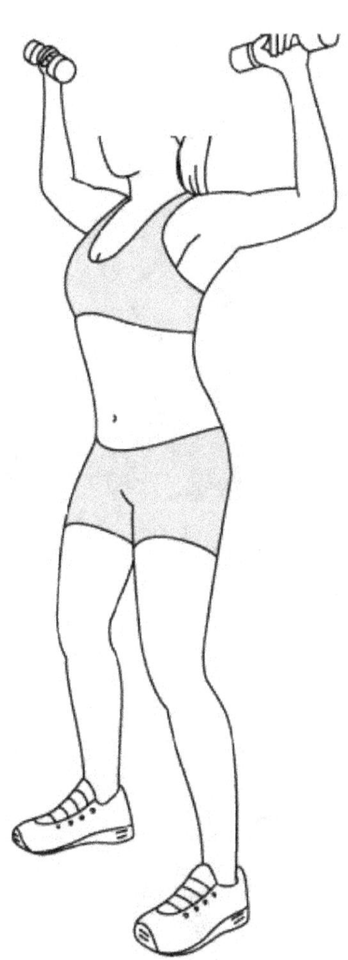

WORKOUT SESSION 2 BACK & SHOULDERS

BACK: 6 exercises / 4 sets / 8 - 10 Reps to Failure.

45/60 Seconds of Rest between Sets

Exercise # 1

Pull Down Elbows Open

Exercise # 2

Pull Down Inverse Grip

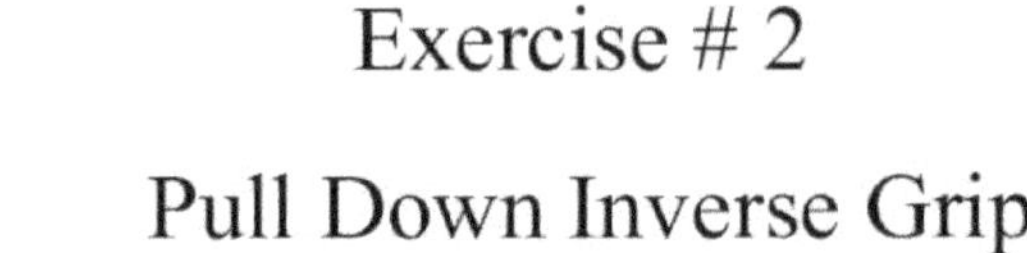

Exercise # 3

Choose one of these Exercises

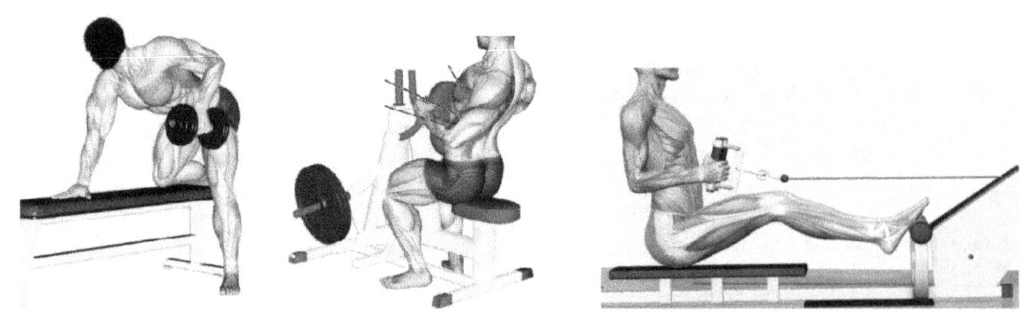

Exercise # 4

Cable Pull Down Straight Harms

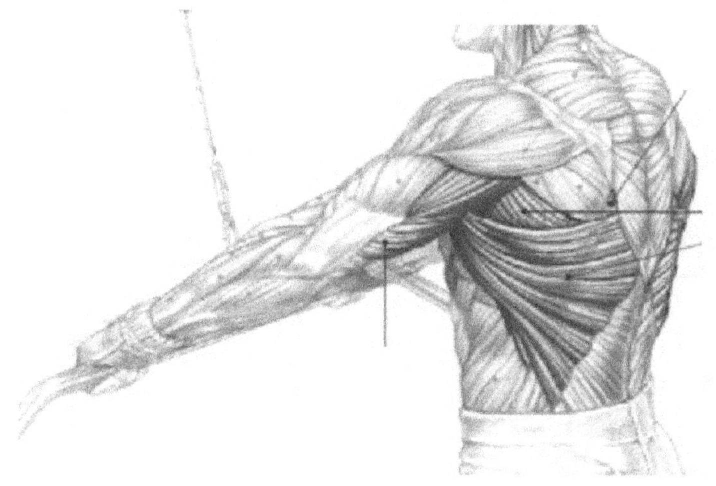

Exercise # 5

Cable Crossover or Machine Revolting Grip

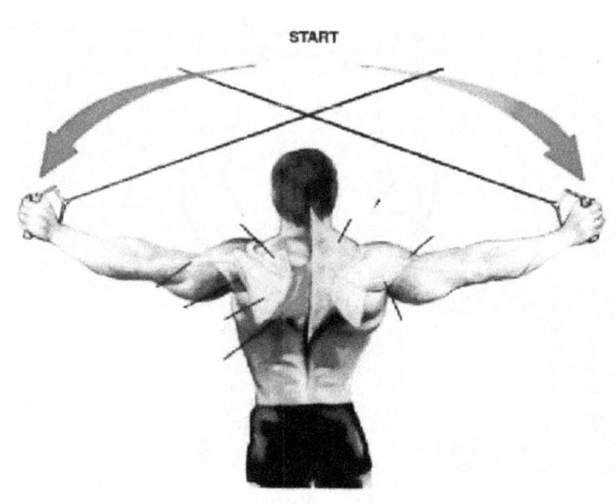

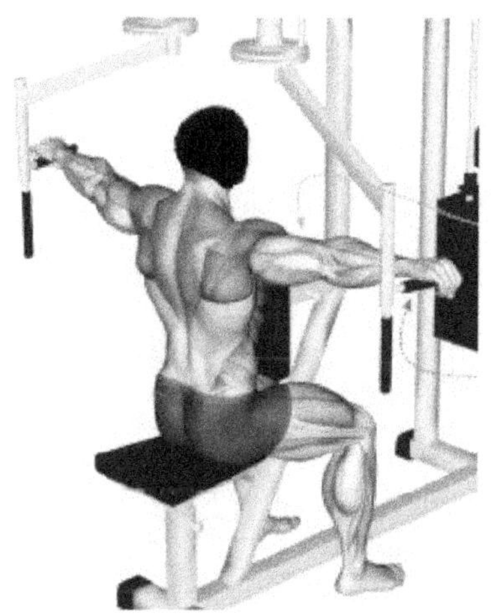

Exercise # 6

With Dumbbells or Barbell

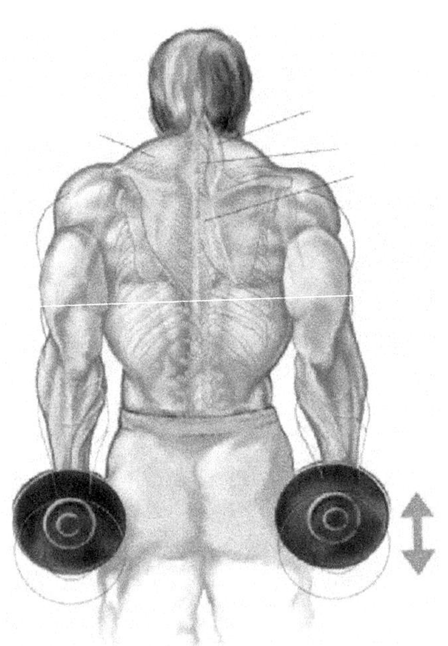

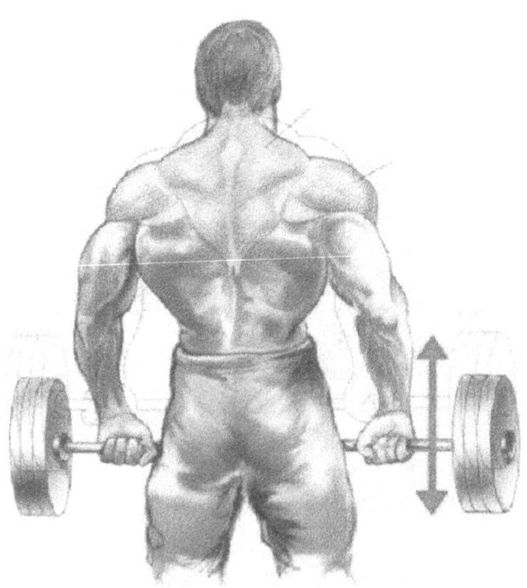

WORKOUT SESSION 3 BICEPS & TRICEPS

BICEPS: 4 Exercises / 4 sets / 8 - 10 Reps to Failure,

45/60 Seconds of Rest between Sets

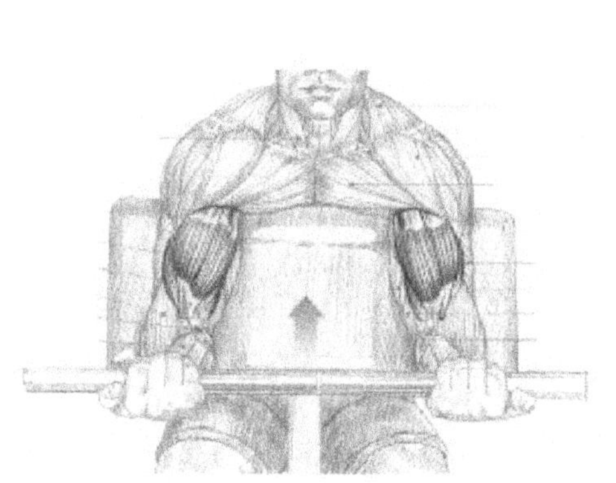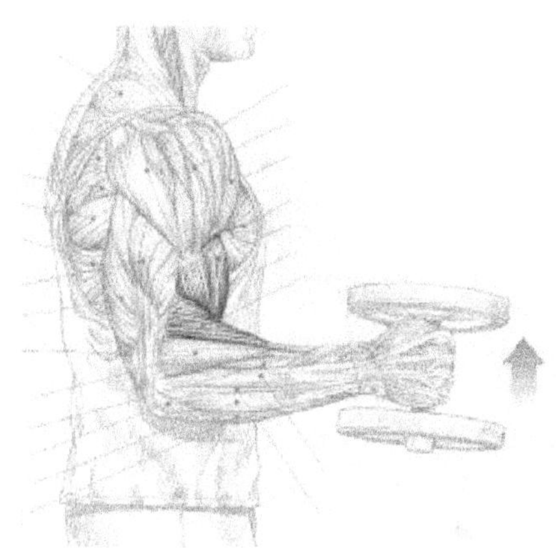

Inverse Grip (picture below)

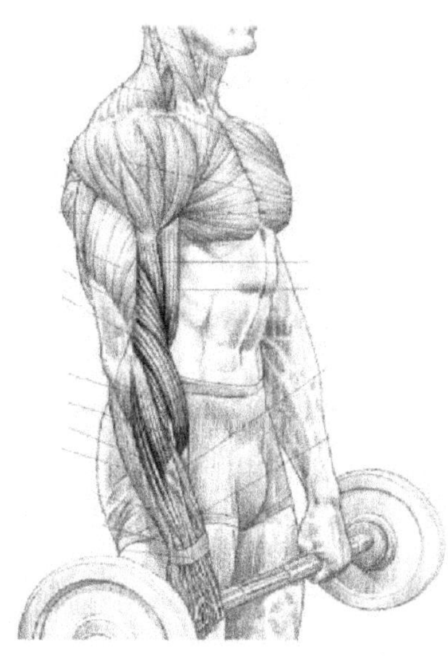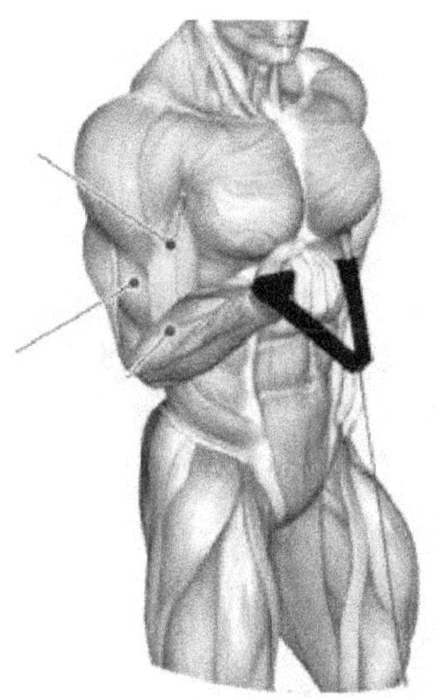

TRICEPS: 4 Exercises / 4 sets / 8 - 10 Reps to Failure

45/60 Seconds of Rest between Sets

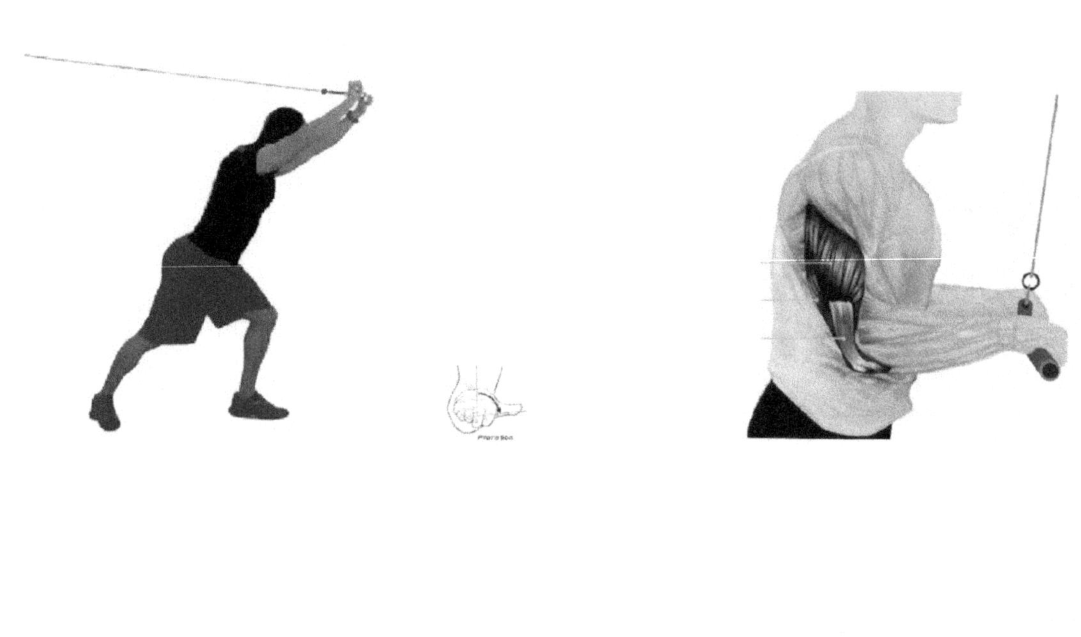

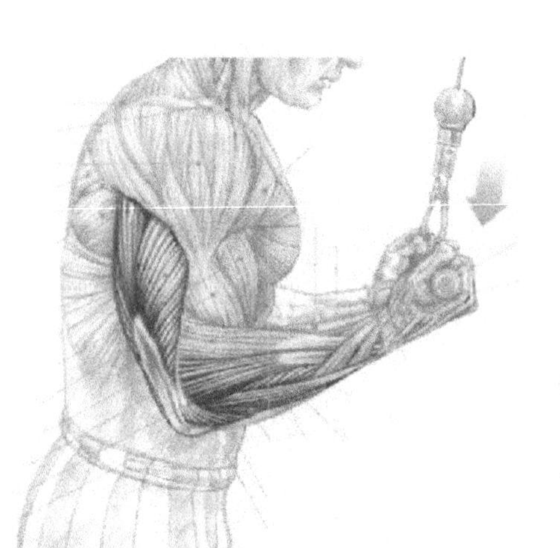

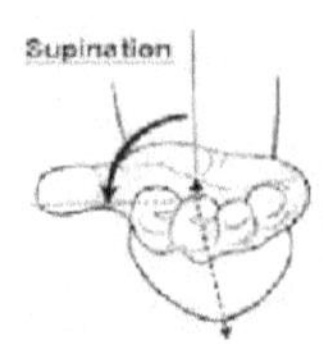

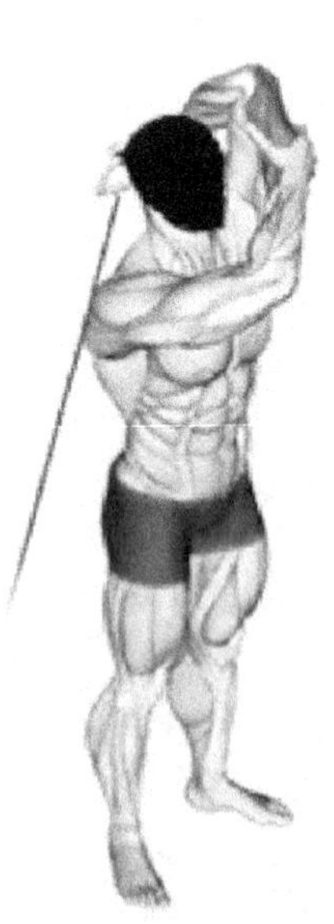

WORKOUT SESSION 4 LEGS

LEGS: 5 Exercises / 4 sets / 8 - 10 Reps to Failure,

45/60 Seconds of Rest between Sets

Both Legs Press

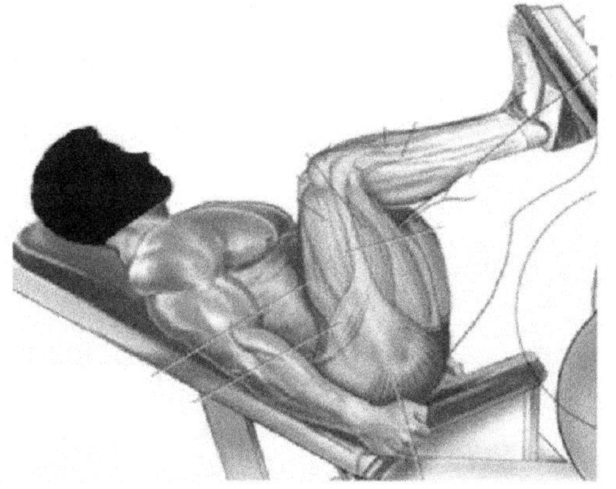

Single Alternate

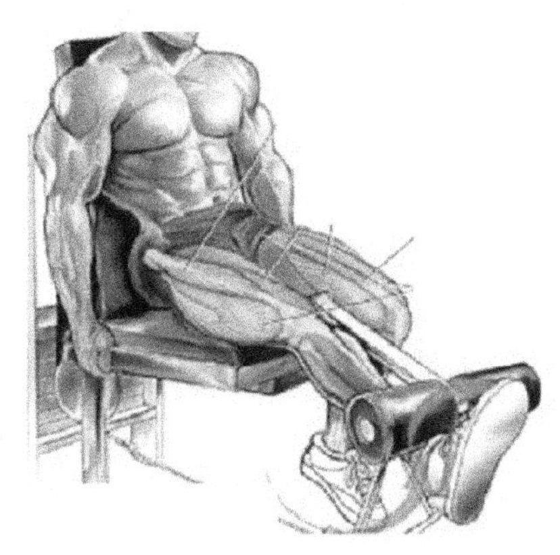

Legs Curl

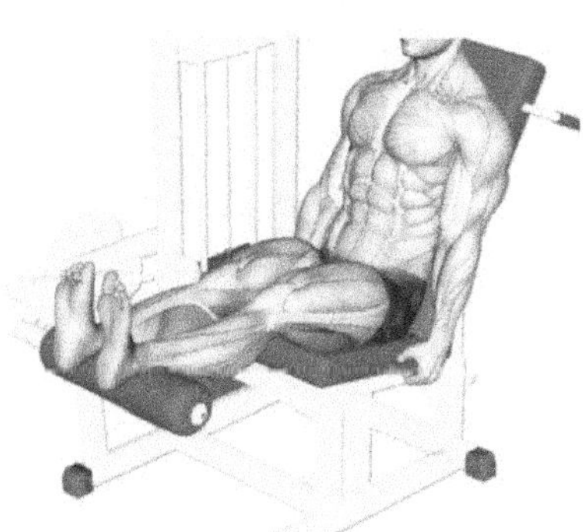

Short Range to Failure

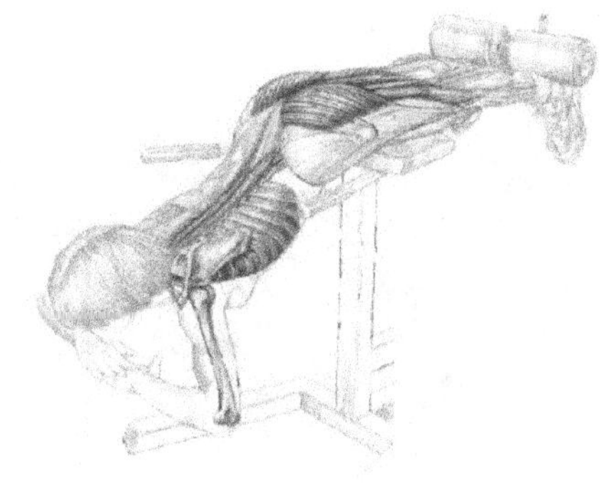

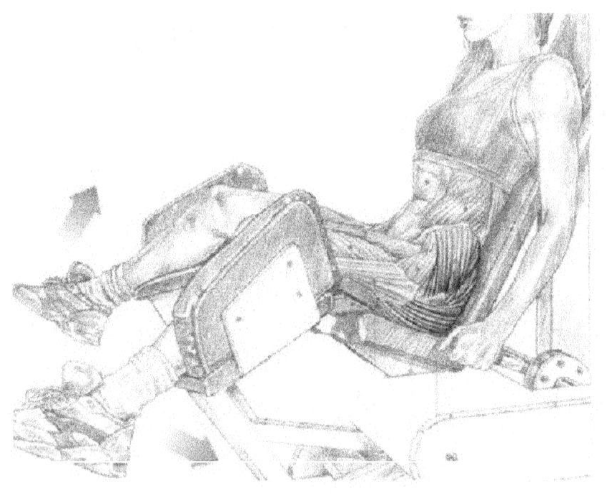

Hip Abduction

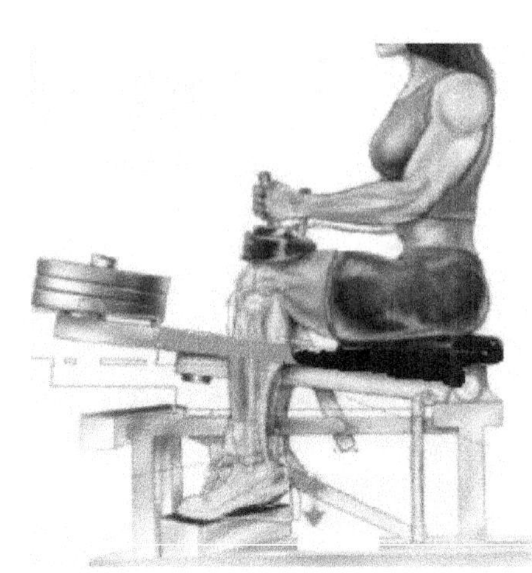

Calf

Calf Exercises Multiple Option Machines

6 Sets, 10 – 15 Reps to Failure

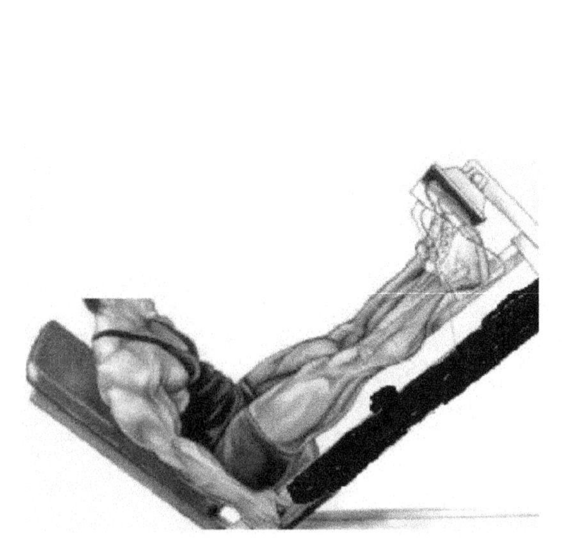

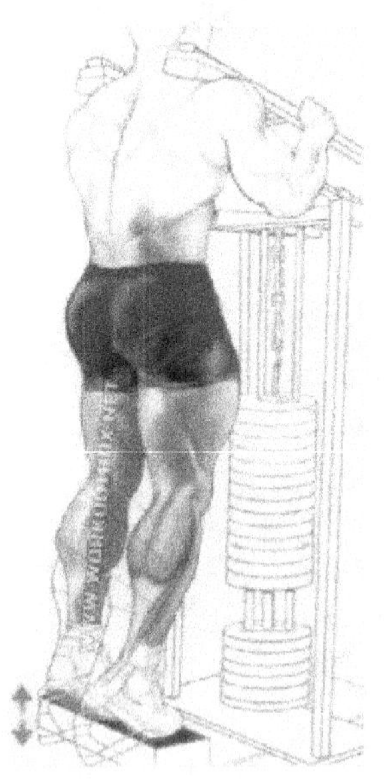

CORE

Tansversus
abdominis
Obliquus internis
abdominis
Obliquus externus
abdominis
Rectus abdominis

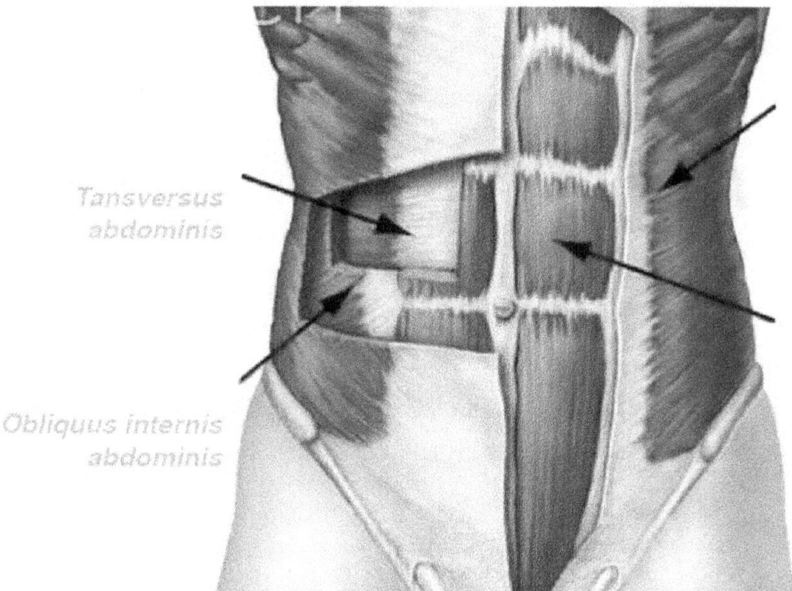

4 Exercises. 1 Exercise per Session at the End. 5 Sets.

As Many As You Can (chose one exercise)

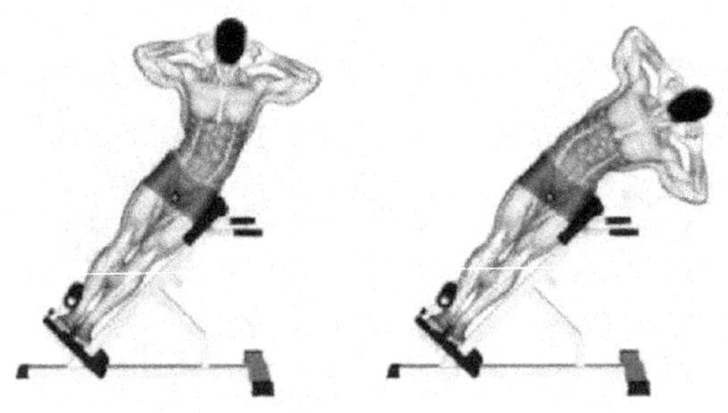

10 Reps to Failure

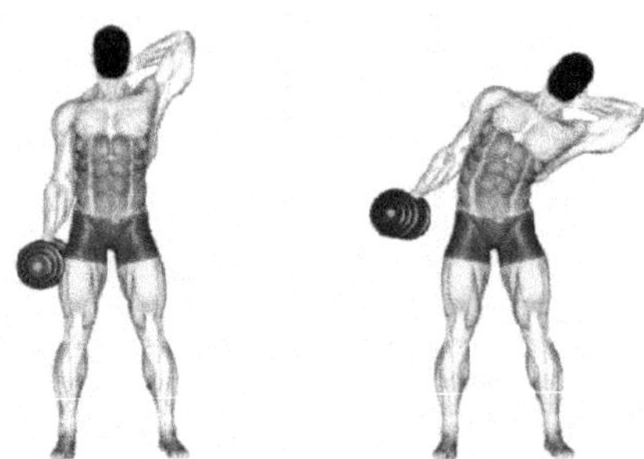

Transverse Cable 10 RPS to Failure

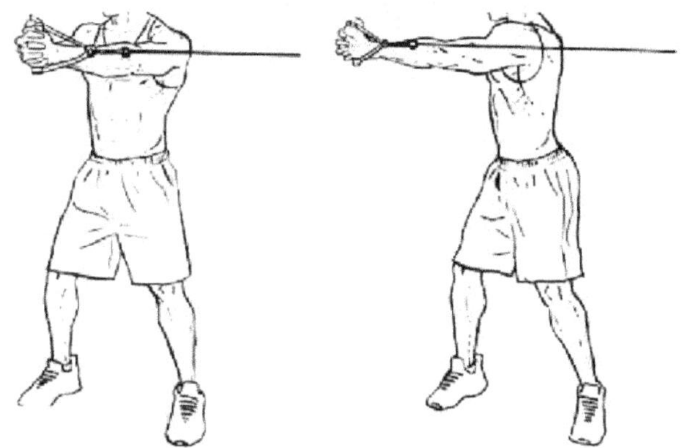

Lower ABS as Many as You Can

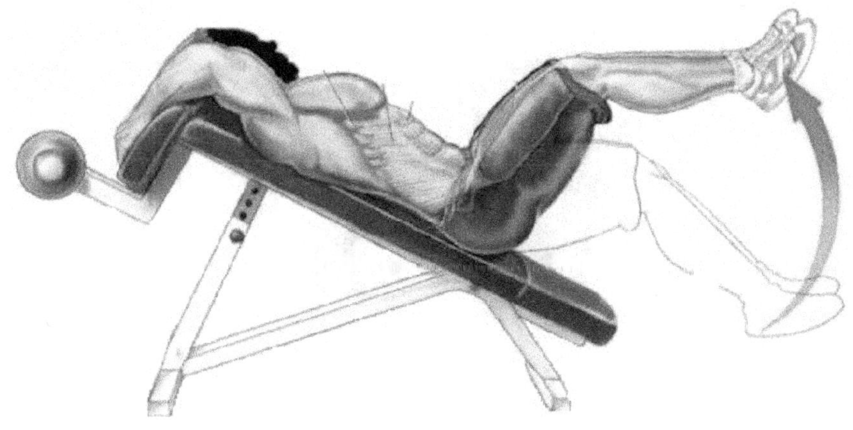

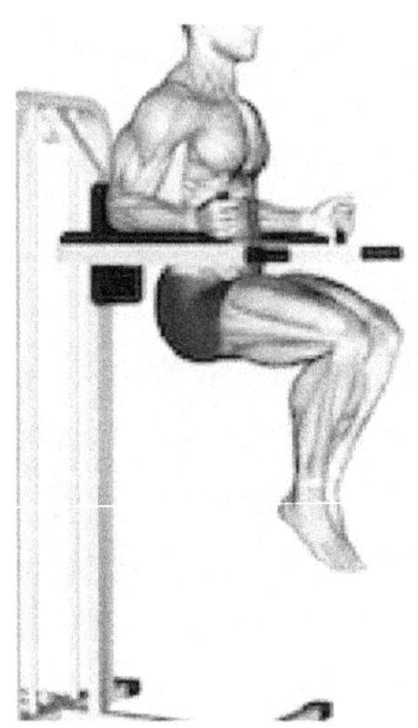

Crunches

10 to15 Reps to Failure to Failure

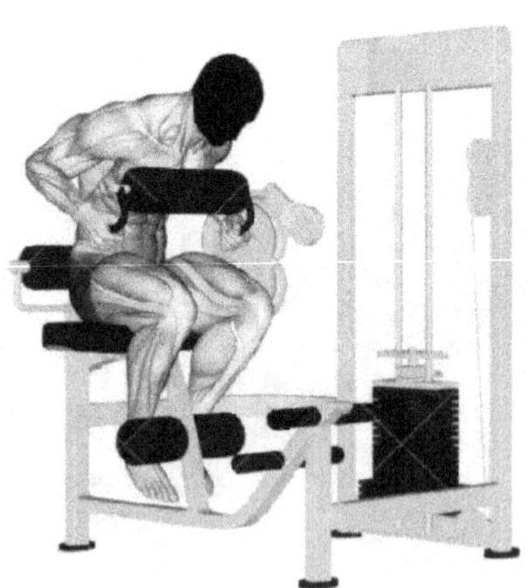

To Failure

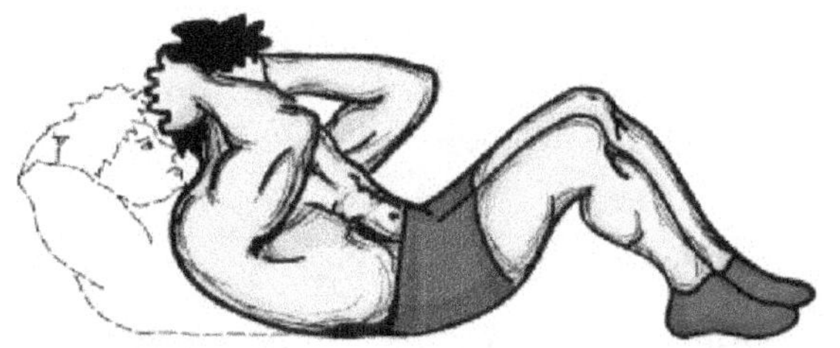

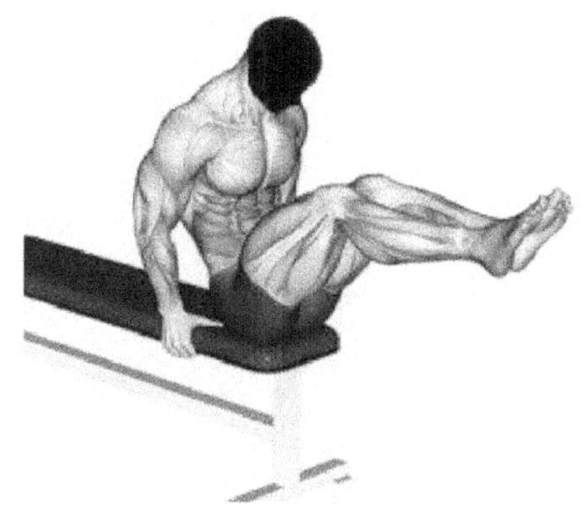

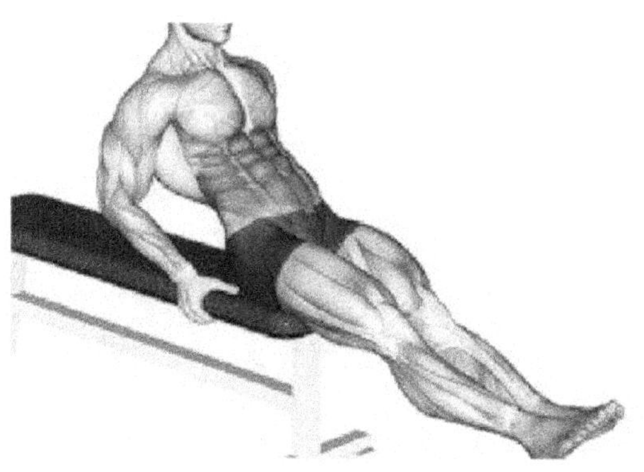

FINAL WORDS

**Paolo Nana is an expert in the fitness world.
His broad education in fitness training and years of experience as a trainer makes him a specialist in the field.**

Among his achievements in the world of bodybuilding, the most known is the title of Mr. Italy. His experience has helped hundreds of people to improve their physical shape. Now you too can learn his method and develop a better body.

I hope this program will help you to improve your overall wellness.

<u>Where there's a will there's a way.</u>

Good luck.

A feedback is always welcome.

<u>paolonanafitness.facebook.com</u>